Heal Yourself: Drug-Free Healing By the Power of New Science & Ancient Wisdom

Phyllis Reardon, M Ed

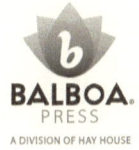

BALBOA
PRESS

A DIVISION OF HAY HOUSE

Phyllis is also the author of Life Coaching Activities & Powerful Questions (2009), Know Your Strengths Inventory (2011), and Life Coaching Questions (2012).

This is a self-help book and as such is not intended to replace your regular health care.

Photo by Beth Kelly Photography

Balboa Press books may be ordered through booksellers or by contacting:

Balboa Press
A Division of Hay House
1663 Liberty Drive
Bloomington, IN 47403
www.balboapress.com
1 (877) 407-4847

Because of the dynamic nature of the Internet, any web addresses or links contained in this book may have changed since publication and may no longer be valid. The views expressed in this work are solely those of the author and do not necessarily reflect the views of the publisher, and the publisher hereby disclaims any responsibility for them.

The author of this book does not dispense medical advice or prescribe the use of any technique as a form of treatment for physical, emotional, or medical problems without the advice of a physician, either directly or indirectly. The intent of the author is only to offer information of a general nature to help you in your quest for emotional and spiritual well-being. In the event you use any of the information in this book for yourself, which is your constitutional right, the author and the publisher assume no responsibility for your actions.

Any people depicted in stock imagery provided by Thinkstock are models, and such images are being used for illustrative purposes only.
Certain stock imagery © Thinkstock.

Printed in the United States of America.

ISBN: 978-1-4525-8623-6 (sc)
ISBN: 978-1-4525-8625-0 (hc)
ISBN: 978-1-4525-8624-3 (e)
Library of Congress Control Number: 2013920455

Balboa Press rev. date: 01/31/2014

Each one of us is totally linked
with the Universe and with all
of life. The Power is within us
to expand the horizons of our
consciousness.

—Louise L. Hay

CONTENTS

PREFACE

This book reveals how Louise Hay healed me.

This is a book of life. It shows how our bodies are *truly us*.

This book shows that good health can be as easy as having a chat.

This book illustrates that we are one with the universe, and that our power comes from the universe, the source. It demonstrates the general knowledge of, ask and you will receive.

In retrospect, knowing what I now know about our life's energy and the connectedness in the world, I know Louise Hay sent energy to me so that I, too, could offer healing to others.

As you read my three stories, you will see how I came to understand what Louise Hay taught me and how it became a part of my being. Now as a certified emotional freedom technique (EFT) practitioner, I continue to offer (in my way) what I learned many years ago from the guru of energy healing, Louise Hay.

I hope that as you read you too will take this information, make it your own, and heal yourself.

This is in part the psychology of how and why self-healing happens. Louise Hay instinctively knew this. I believe she was placed here to direct as many of us as possible to the healing path.

Twenty years ago, this amazing woman understood what she had to tell the world, and tell the world she did.

I only hope I continue to attract and lead people on this healing path. In Part I, I share my stories of self-healing. In Part II, I give the science behind the healing in self-healing and how it can work for you. And in Part III, I share the language I used, and continue to use, to heal myself through body-chat scripts.

ACKNOWLEDGMENTS

The universe has been very generous to me over the years. It has offered me an amazing life. Because of this amazement and wonder, I understood I could heal myself.

The universe has sent me many kind and loving people along my life's journey, Louise Hay being one of the most powerful. Thank you, Louise.

Thank you to my family for your encouragement, especially my husband, Tom.

Thank you to my team of readers who kindly offered support and editing advise.

PART I

My Stories of Self-Healing

ഇ൬ൽ

How I Met Louise Hay

Born with Positivity

I was always a positive person. I got that from my parents. They lived through the Great Depression, and life was not always easy for them. But despite their hardships, they decided to view each day in a positive light, for which I am grateful. This skill of positivity I learned well from them.

Happiness and love filled my early development days, and I have taken that forward into my adult life. This is important for me to state up front, as the focus of this book deals with how you as an individual perceive the world—your mind-set. This book reflects my experiences, and in sharing them, I hope that you and those you love will benefit in a positive, healthy way.

The system I use comes from different teachings and techniques. I have been a student of the universe. I have listened. I have learned. I have experienced. I have developed a process that works for me. As you read, please make note of what speaks to you. Take what worked for me, and make it your own.

I always see the glass as half full and days as sunny with few clouds. That does not mean you have to be super positive to make my technique work, but a little tilt toward the positive side of things certainly helps.

It is important for me to note that positivity is a skill. It needs to be worked on and helps build the mind-set in which you view the world. Positive Mental Attitude (PMA) and mind-set are essential to understanding yourself and your health.

Self-healing came to me as much from my intuition—my body's voice—as it did from real-life experiences. What do people generally say? Experience is the best teacher. Unfortunately, many times the lessons we learn come from difficult situations. It makes me wonder if the lessons learned from pleasant happenings are as dramatic in our cognitive shifts; I am sure there is a body of research somewhere on this very topic.

I would now like to share with you how my life experiences shaped my thinking, perception, and mind-set in relation to conventional medicine.

My Son's Near-Death Experience

In 1974, I was a young mother of two delightful little boys, a four-year-old and a one-year-old. My four-year-old son, Sean, was born with what doctors told me was an outward-draining cyst located on the side of his head near the temple area. In time, they explained, this would grow over and disappear.

That summer, while on a fishing trip with his dad, my son was bitten by a mosquito in the area of the cyst. A trip to the hospital resulted in an outpatient visit to remove the cyst. This simple procedure turned into a life-altering event for the whole family.

Two craniotomies and nine years later, my son was finally released from one of the leading neurological surgeons in North America. One doctor's error had to be corrected by another but not without many stressful years for our family.

This was my doorway to questioning what at that point I accepted as an infallible institution. I believe now that the culture and society in which I grew up, one of a strong Catholic faith, discouraged any questioning. My perception of education was "Don't question but accept all authority on blind faith."

My life experiences changed that. It took the near-death of my first child to shake me into the reality and the humanness of our health care providers.

At the age of twenty-seven, I began to question. I began looking at my health and the health of my children with more responsibility. I think as a mother I instinctively did this, but it became more ingrained in me to look at alternatives to our accepted medical system. I guess my personal experiences caused me to lose faith to some degree. Loss of faith brings with it a bit of bitterness, but I had to learn to release that.

This is the backdrop for what was to become a new way of my perceiving and caring for my physical body. It was also my first step onto the path that led me to Louise Hay.

During this experience with my son—the many trips to the hospital, his long stays, waiting outside the operating room during lengthy surgeries, the sounds and smells of the intensive care unit, watching the surgeon approach after each surgery and trying to read his expression—I did my very best to stay positive. I would talk to myself in a positive way. Not once did I allow a negative, imagined end result enter my mind, not even when the neurologist in his surgery greens approached with worry beads rotating on his fingers. I focused on a future of hope and health, a future filled with fun activities for my then five-year-old son.

When Sean left the hospital for the final time, I had to learn to mother with caution but not paralysis. I could not let this physical condition control him or me. I listened to my inner voice, and he was on ice skates one month out of the hospital, a dream he had during his long hospital stay.

The technique I used to stay positive at that time was self-talk, but I did not use that phrase then. I do not think I had any label on what I did. I think I just knew that when I spoke to myself in a positive way, I would feel better. When I visualized a positive outcome, I truly believed it would happen. My son now lives a healthy, activity-filled life and works in the holistic personal health arena. And to this day, he plays ice hockey twice a week.

I have been in tune with my body since my mid-twenties. I am intuitive, so maybe that allows me to be more in tune with my body as I listen to it. Whether it is intuition, bodily instinct, or another term, one thing I am sure of is I have healed myself. I have done this on at least three separate occasions. I feel so strongly about this healing process that I want to share it with as many people as possible. Even though my health issues were common to women, this healing technique can be used by both genders of all ages.

Birth and Life Perspective

My life began in the midst of a winter blizzard so severe that my mother's doctor did not make it to the hospital. On that extremely snowy day of January 3, 1947, the only doctor available at our hospital was an orthopedic specialist. He delivered me.

Having given birth to four wonderful, healthy children, I sometimes wonder how the birthing process influences each individual's unique life path. On that day in January 1947, a discussion undoubtedly happened at my mother's bedside around this most unlikely physician performing my delivery. Possibly, this discussion in some way embedded on my subconscious and informed me to consider alternatives, as this indeed was an alternative delivery.

6

Did my experience then, both in the womb and during delivery, inform and form my alternative health decisions in later life? Although my life started in 1947, the healing stories I am about to tell you began in the 1980s.

All of my children were born in the seventies: 1970, 1973, 1976, and 1978. I was blessed with four healthy, wonderful children—three handsome sons and one beautiful daughter. Following the 1978 birth of my youngest son, I decided it was time to get fit. Four pregnancies had constituted thirty-six months—a combined three years—of my life, so it was time to get my body back in shape. And that I did. The YMCA fit the bill. I not only worked out there, I also became one of their fitness instructors. I was feeling really healthy!

By the autumn of 1988 and into the winter of 1989, I began experiencing what for me were abnormal monthly menstrual periods. And at forty-two, I struggled on a monthly basis with physical pain during my periods. My life at this time was extremely busy. Not only was I a mother of four, but I was also working full-time as an assistant director of an alternate high school for disenfranchised inner-city youth. My mom had passed in 1987, my last surviving parent, and I missed her. Many emotions filled me.

My menstrual problems increased. Along with the intensity and lengthened duration of my period came severe physical pain and discomfort. This was a new paradigm in my personal health. My body had never experienced this before.

The pain moved me so far outside my comfort zone and my usual health regime that I resorted to taking over-the-counter painkillers. Topping out between eight and ten painkillers a day, this by a person who got drowsy after taking a single aspirin, made me realize there was something seriously wrong, something that needed the attention of my family doctor.

Based on my symptoms, my family doctor strongly recommended I see a gynecologist. With a degree of frustration—I am not sure why, as my past gynecologist had been a brilliant male physician—I asked if I could see a female gynecologist.

Maybe it was my forty-two-year-old feminist exerting her power and finding her place in my world. Maybe I was at a point in my life where I just wanted someone who could fully understand what it was like to have a uterus, a well-worked womb, a special female body part. Maybe, just maybe I did not want some male commenting, "You have four kids. You don't need your womb anymore."

I wanted a doctor who understood that this special body part meant more to a woman than as a baby machine. The uterus plays a large role in blood flow for sexual stimulation, which for me was part of how I defined myself as a woman. It was psychological. I had no intention of giving up this body part without a fight or at least some strong discussion.

For whatever reason, I made my request, and my family doctor was fully supportive. He referred me to a woman who he said was the best around. However, she practiced outside our city in a town that was over two-hours driving time.

Mid-February was appointment day, and in eastern Canada that means snow-covered, icy roads at best. Having prepared the kids' meals for that day, arranged child care, and taken an annual leave day, I headed out over the wintry highway with my husband. I did not want anyone to know, so I told the kids I had a meeting out of town, which I think goes under the category of "white lie," as I *was* meeting with someone.

On reflection, I do not recall much about the drive out, but I certainly will never forget the drive back. But I am getting ahead of myself, which I tend to do some times.

It was a cold, damp, dull Friday morning as we entered the town of Clarenville, Newfoundland. The red-brick building was easy to find. The half-empty hospital parking lot with its small piles of snow gave a sense of a not-too-busy day. As usual, I maintained my positive attitude.

The hospital smell and shiny floors that greeted us as we entered made my heart flutter just a little. The realization set in that in all my visits to the hospital to see my son fifteen years prior, this hospital visit was all about me. But I remained positive. Phyllis, the eternal optimist!

The waiting room was uninviting, but then who really wants to be invited into a hospital? The green faux-leather chairs with their chrome legs offered no solace, but I was determined to stay the positive course.

I am not sure how long we waited, but it was indeed a relief, if you can feel relief when waiting to see a gynecologist, when my name was called.

I was delighted that this very professional female doctor with a wonderful British accent oozed confidence while having the ability to put me at ease.

She read my chart, and after a few regular questions, my feet were secured in metal stirrups, and she began her examination of my forty-two-year-old, very-productive body part. Immediately following the procedure, she had me wait in her office and asked my husband to join us.

Minutes passed. Then she entered, holding my folder. She looked somewhat more serious but still comforting. As she began speaking, I felt as though I were transported to another time, sitting and watching a movie in a foreign language. The words that came from her mouth were directed at me, but I was sure they were intended for someone else. I now know I went into slight shock when I heard her say, "You have a large tumor in your uterus, and you need a hysterectomy as soon as possible. I can do the surgery at this hospital, but I am suggesting you be better served by being in your own city close to family."

I do not remember how I left her office. Did I say thank you? Did I even shake her hand? I do not know.

Positivity Left Me

Hospital? Surgery? Not Phyllis! She is too healthy!

As my husband drove our burgundy 1987 Chrysler out of the hospital parking lot and onto the byway, I began to cry. Tears rolled down my cheeks, and my stomach felt queasy. My heart hurt for me and for my family. To my current knowledge, a tumor meant one thing: cancer. I felt physically sick.

The distance from the hospital parking lot along the byway to the highway is about half a mile. I felt the car slow as it came to the stop sign. I looked up. There in big red letters on the weather-beaten, octagon-shaped sign was the word *STOP*. It was as if I were hearing a voice in my head shout the word loud and clear. *STOP. Stop your crying. Stop the self-pity. Stop the negative images that are floating in your head. Get a life, Phyllis!*

I immediately grabbed some tissues, wiped away the last tears, and rubbed the sniffles from my nose. That was it. I did not have time to cry. I did not have time for self-pity. I had four children ranging in age from eleven to nineteen who needed me. They needed me in the way they were used to having their mom—healthy, positive, and full of energy. I needed to *heal my body*.

By the time we pulled away from the stop sign and onto the highway for our trip home, my tears and self-pity were abated. Positivity was back, albeit not 100 percent, maybe not even 40 percent. But it was there, gaining strength with every icy mile we covered.

I needed a plan—not sure what kind of a plan—but I knew I needed one. My thoughts went back to fifteen years earlier and how I dealt with the health scare of my oldest son. I remembered that I talked to myself in a kind way and did not allow myself to imagine a negative result for him. I now decided to do the same for myself. Negative endings were not an option. I had to get well.

My thoughts turned to my uterus. You already understand how I feel about this precious body part. It defined me, provided pleasure, and protected my children in gestational days. It was an integral part of who Phyllis was. The question "How do I keep it?" flooded my mind.

Meeting Louise Hay

The next day was a Saturday, and many chores for a working mom of four waited for completion. But on this mom's mind was her healing. The self-help industry had not yet taken off at that time, at least not to the extent that it has in more recent years. I failed to mention that I am an educator and a bit of an academic, so I have a tendency to turn to books for answers. We were pre-Google in 1989, so I needed to find my answers in paper and ink.

Late that Saturday afternoon, between music lessons and hockey games, I headed to my neighborhood bookstore. I was not exactly sure what to look for, but something or someone made me feel I would find just the right book for my needs. It may have been that voice that screamed at me at the stop sign.

I went directly to the self-help section, which at that time was limited. In fact, this was my first time in the self-help section.

I moved slowly from book cover to book cover. Within a short time, I saw this little blue book with the words *Heal Your Body* printed on the cover. *This has to be the book. These are the exact words that came into my mind at that stop sign,* I thought to myself. Now here it was, written right on the cover of a published book. I am not sure what words I used at that moment to express myself, but by today's vernacular, I would have said, "How good is that!" or "Now that's what I'm talking about!"

I examined the book, checked the publication date, publication city, author, and did a quick perusal of the book. It felt right in my hands.

In the narrow aisle of the self-help section of my local bookstore, I met Louse Hay.

That night, my bedtime reading was Louise Hay's *Heal Your Body*. I remember that each time I went through the process that Louise recommended, I had this overpowering feeling that this wonderful woman wrote this book just for me. How could she possibly know what I needed? I felt the connection.

Now this was a tool, and tools only work if they are utilized. So on that cold Saturday night in February 1989, I began my self-healing journey. Each time I did my self-healing session, I could feel Louise Hay right there in the room with me. I now believe she was, as we are all connected in the universe.

As I became familiar with Louise's process, I would add other parts and words that came to my mind. I was faithful to my self-healing process. Every day for at least three times a day, seven days a week, I would practice self-healing as suggested by Louise Hay.

I would take the golden light from the universe, have it enter the crown of my head, and have it flow gently through my body until it got to my womb. I would then visualize the tumor in my uterus as being red and raw. I would then surround my uterus with this golden universal light and watch as the redness and rawness disappeared. I watched as my uterus healed.

I began adding my own thoughts to the process that Louise Hay taught me. I talked to my uterus, telling it how important it was to me. I told it that I needed to stay healthy for my four children.

Day in, day out, I was faithful to my self-healing routine. And Louise Hay was with me on my healing path.

Hysterectomy?

I should mention that after my return from the appointment with the female gynecologist in Clarenville, I met with my family doctor for an appointment with a local gynecologist who was to perform the needed hysterectomy. Remember that was suggested so I could be close to my family while I had the needed surgery?

It took three months to get an appointment with this next doctor, a relatively short time period for a specialist, as the request had been labeled urgent.

I was consistent with my self-healing sessions for the next three months. Louise Hay was with me every day. With her words in my head, not once did I stray from my healing routine. It is most important that I mention I strongly believed I could heal myself, and that I fully intended to have this tumor gone from my body. Later, I will elaborate on these two concepts: belief and intention.

To this point, I had not told my children. In fact, when they read this book, this will be news to them.

The day came for my appointment. I had asked my family doctor for an unbiased examination. The visit was treated somewhat as a second opinion, so previous results were not shared at that time.

For the second time in three months, I found myself in stirrups on a cold, metal examination table. After the thorough internal exam was complete, I was surprised to hear this male doctor say that all was good.

I looked at him strangely and asked, "Don't I have a tumor? Are you sure I don't have a tumor?"

He replied matter-of-factly, "All feels really good to me. No tumor. You have a healthy uterus."

Well, so much for my insistence on a female gynecologist, I thought. *A lot she knew!*

Family Doctor's Wisdom

Within two days, I was sitting in the familiar, soft-black leather chair in my family doctor's office, as follow-up was needed. As he entered his office, these words immediately spilled from my mouth, "Well, I guess you were wrong about Dr. Female Gyno being one of the best around. She was wrong on this one. She diagnosed a tumor in my uterus, and this doctor clearly stated that I have a healthy womb."

My younger-but-wiser family doctor looked at me and slowly and deliberately asked, "What have you been doing for the past three months Phyllis?"

I had not told him I was religiously doing self-healing, but he must have sensed it. I hesitated and then responded, "I've been practicing self-healing three times a day every day for the past three months."

As slowly and deliberately as he had asked the question, he said, "Well, Phyllis, you have obviously healed yourself."

I did? Could this be correct? Could I actually have healed myself? I know I believed I could. Did I truly accomplish it?

I did! My kids will have their mom for a long time. I healed myself! Every cell in my body echoed joy.

Amazing stuff! The kind of thing you want to shout from the rooftops, but this was 1989, so who would have listened? Who would have believed me? On several occasions, I brought up the topic only to get an uncomfortable reaction from my listener. The reaction when you know you are not believed. So I stopped telling my story.

My self-healing was one of the most amazing experiences in my life up to that time. Louise Hay received a special "thank you" from me daily. I sang her praises and shared her book. What she taught me stayed with me. She saved my life. She returned a healthy mom back to her four children.

I continued practicing what I learned from Louise Hay. I took it and made it mine, but it was Louise Hay who got me on my way along the path of self-healing.

Lessons Learned from Louise Hay

Louise Hay taught me that I had the power to heal myself.

Louise Hay taught me that I could speak to my body parts and they would indeed listen.

Louise Hay taught me that I needed to converse with my body daily.

Louise Hay taught me to listen to my body.

Louise Hay taught me a life-altering technique.

Louise Hay taught me to ask and I shall receive.

Louise Hay taught me that I am part of a greater force.

Story One: Conclusion

Through these lessons I learned from Louise Hay, I approached the rest of my health.

Equipped with this new knowledge and skills to self-heal and communicate with my body, I experienced yet another amazing self-healing. The following tells the story.

Louise Hay planted the seeds for my body chats. This woman who I had not met came into my mind each time I did them. I felt as though she were there with me, giving me energy for this alternative way of healing. I felt as if she were saying to me, "Take the knowledge I have given you and expand it into the future."

I did.

ଞ୦ଓଃ

Who Knew They Were Listening?

This is another of my life-healing stories that shows the power of communicating with your body and the power of belief and intention.

I would like you to stop reading now and reflect for a moment on how you talk to your body.

I often say in my workshops that if we spoke to friends the way we spoke to our self, we would spend most of our time alone. What do you say about your hair, nose, teeth, skin, butt, or waist?

Imagine if you would. You plan to meet your best friend for coffee at your favorite coffee shop, and as he or she approaches, you say, "Susie, what a mess your hair is today!" or "Joe, when did your gut get that big?" I am guessing that after that you would be sipping that java all by yourself.

For women reading this, please reflect on the words you use as the time of the month approaches for your monthly period. You know the words I am talking about.

Make a mental list of some comments you make about your menstrual cycle. The negative comments and terms used to describe this natural process for many are grounded in our culture. It is what we heard from female members of our family and friends and the media. Some of these expressions are not at all complimentary to the uterus. Terms I recall hearing are: on the rag, curse of Dracula, ugly red aunt, leak week, and hated monthly visitor. None of these are endearing terms to say the least!

Your Uterus

This is your uterus, performing its natural task, providing hormones to keep you healthy. It is a part of your body's process. Your uterus is you. It has helped define you. If you are a biological mom, it gave you your children. If you are an adoptive mom, your child was held in a uterus while waiting your arrival. If you are a surrogate mom, your uterus provided a sanctuary for another's child to grow. Yet when it performs its main purpose, releasing unused eggs, its amazing well-calculated function, you get upset with it. You complain. You speak to your uterus unkindly. You call it nasty names.

Most of us at some time are verbally abusive to our own bodies. Why then are we so surprised when they revolt? The bodily revolution shows up as pain, discomfort, off-balance body energy, disease, and a myriad of other health issues. Have you ever thought that maybe, just maybe, if you were nicer to your body parts they would reciprocate?

Reactive to Proactive Healing

I learned well from Louise Hay the power we have to heal our bodies. I took what I learned from Louise and created for myself my own body chats. From 1989, when I first discovered Louise Hay, and for ten years forward, I occasionally spoke to my body parts, mostly if I encountered pain or discomfort. I guess I used my technique at that time in a reactive manner. If something went wrong, I took to self-healing body chats to help correct the imbalance in my body.

This all changed the summer of 1999.

Ten years had passed since my discovery of Louise Hay's book *Heal Your Body*. I had continued on an as-needed basis to self-heal through my body chats, but the story I am about to relate changed all that.

It was July 1999, and I was attending a Multiple Intelligence Institute at Harvard University. However, due to lack of dorm space, we were housed on the campus of Tufts University.

This institute, under the direction of Dr. Howard Gardner, was, to say the least, an intense ten days of research, study, and learning. By design, halfway through, we were given a free day to catch up on studies, writing, or shopping, or to just relax. I chose the latter, as I had already had the Boston shopping experience.

Another reason I chose to relax and read that day was I had just started my menstrual period. I was now fifty-two years old and had been having regular monthly periods, nothing unusual albeit a little heavier over the past year.

If you have not been to Tufts campus, it is a very relaxing place, especially in July. I walked, reflected, and reflected some more.

My dorm consisted of one very narrow bunk bed, a well-worn desk with multiple fonts of engraved initials, a wooden chair, and three twisted wire clothes hangers in a doorless closet. Nothing to distract the mind.

Mid-afternoon, I retreated to my room as much to escape the heat as to rest and reflect some more. My thoughts turned to my uterus; yes, my womb. My mind was completely focused on it. What was happening? These thoughts had not occurred to me before.

Questions about my uterus floated in and out of my head. *How long have we been together? What functions have you played in my life? Do you ever talk to me? Do you know my children? Do you have a connection to my children?*

The questions started spinning in my head. I have no idea why my thoughts went in this direction. Yes, I was having my period, but that had been happening for the past thirty-six years, and I had not experienced those thoughts before. Sure, I spoke to my uterus if I had discomfort. I spoke to it on an as-needed basis to release pain, but that was it. I was not intimate with it. Yet at that moment, as I sat in that sparse room, I was filled with the feeling that my uterus was not just a body part but also a person, a human entity, someone who had been with me on my life's journey.

I decided right there and then to write a salute to my womb. I thought I would give it a humorous twist. I started to write.

Upon my colleague's return from her shopping expedition, she dropped by my room to show me her newly purchased treasures and to see how I spent my day. I related how my day went, and when I got to the part about writing an amusing salute to my uterus, she was very interested in hearing it. I obliged her by reading my uterus salute to her.

When I finished, to my surprise, my poem had had the opposite effect. Tears were flowing down her cheeks as she said, "This is not funny. This is heavy."

At first, I was disappointed, as I had failed in my first attempt to write an amusing poem. I am not sure why I thought it was light and funny, as I am not a harsh person. I guess I was coming from a place of happiness and not humor when I wrote this salute to my womb. It was joy I was expressing.

As I have stated, on that day, my uterus did not feel like it was just a body part but like a person, a human entity, someone who had been with me on my life's journey. I therefore decided to give my womb a human name. I thought a little alliteration would work, so I named my womb Wilma.

The poem Wilma Womb follows on page 22. Maybe you will smile or like my colleague you, too, may shed a tear. However you react, the point is not your reaction but how my body benefited from my writing this poem, or, I should say, from chatting with my womb.

Wilma Womb

Wilma Womb has wasted away
Why, Wilma, now that I have a free day?
A free night, too, what can I do?
Wombless, oh Wilma, what can I do?

> The womb is a very safe place.
> Held my children till I saw their face,
> Saw their face, washed their face,
> Their hands, their feet, and tied their lace.

Wilma Womb has wasted away
Why, Wilma, now that I have a free day?
A free night, too, what can I do?
Wombless, oh Wilma, what can I do?

> My womb has always been a part of me.
> Didn't use it until I was twenty-three.
> Twenty-three, twenty-six, thirty, and thirty-two.
> Oh, Wilma Womb, now what do I do?

Wilma Womb has wasted away
Why, Wilma, now that I have a free day?
A free night, too, what can I do?
Wombless, oh Wilma, what can I do?

> The woes and worries of menopause I have to face.
> Life can be a strange place.
> A strange place 'cause no one said
> The womb you won't have till your dead.

Wilma Womb has wasted away
Why, Wilma, now that I have a free day?
A free night, too, what can I do?
Wombless, oh Wilma, what can I do?

The days they pass, the nights too,
Hot and sweaty, making me blue.
Natural remedies? HRT?
Oh, Wilma, could you advise? What will it be?

Wilma Womb has wasted away
Why, Wilma, now that I have a free day?
A free night, too, what can I do?
Wombless, oh Wilma, what can I do?

It's your age, they advise
Doctors male, female. Are these lies?
Who to ask? What to read?
Grear may not give me a lead.

Wilma Womb has wasted away
Why, Wilma, now that I have a free day?
A free night, too, what can I do?
Wombless, oh Wilma, what can I do?

I guess, Wilma, it's me and you
Back before I was twenty-two.
Twenty-two, thirty-two, forty-two, fifty-two.
We have to decide just what to do.

Wilma Womb has wasted away
Why, Wilma, now that I have a free day?
A free night, too, what can I do?
Wombless, oh Wilma, what can I do?

Surgery or atrophy … we must part.
I tell you this straight from my heart.
You did your job. You did it well.
And many a story, dear Wilma, you allowed me to tell.

Wilma Womb has wasted away
Why, Wilma, now that I have a free day?
A free night, too, what can I do?
Wombless, oh Wilma, what can I do?

You will not be with me as I go forward.
How many more years, I don't know.
But this, dear Wilma, be assured
Your years of service four futures secured.

Wilma Womb has wasted away
Why, Wilma, now that I have a free day?
A free night, too, what can I do?
Wombless, oh Wilma, what can I do?

My period ran its regular number of days and finished the day before I was to head home after a once-in-a-lifetime learning experience at Harvard.

I remember well the day I flew out of Boston Logan Airport. It was July 16, 1999, a beautiful sunny Friday afternoon. *Not a cloud in the sky,* I remember thinking the next day when I heard the news of the fatal plane crash that claimed the life of John F. Kennedy Jr. Some dates never leave us.

That Monday, I was back to work and my regular activities. My scribbled poem was tucked away in the bottom drawer of my file cabinet with the rest of my notes from that brilliant Harvard experience.

Twenty-eight days after my Wilma composition, although never a Girl Guide, I was prepared for my menstrual cycle. I scooted to the local pharmacy to get my needed supply, a well-practiced, thirty-six-year routine. But this turned out to be the period that never was.

Period. Full Stop. I was educated within the British vernacular, and the end of a sentence was never called a period. It was a "full stop," and this is exactly what I experienced.

A full stop? Or was it a pause? I waited. August eased its way into September. September moved along. Pumpkins and witches disappeared from front lawns to be replaced by red and green lights. I still waited.

No more monthly menstruation periods.

During the month of November, as I was doing one of my two-way body chats, I heard a female voice in my head saying, "You gave me permission to finish my work, so I have retired."

At that moment, my thoughts went to the scribbled notes tucked away in my home office. The poem "Wilma Womb." Was this the key to the sudden, unexpected full stop?

I frantically dug through the stacks of paper. There it was, folded and tucked safely inside the pocket of my burgundy Harvard binder. The answer.

The Answer

I had the answer in the words I felt and heard that day, in the belief I had about my womb. I had it in the thoughts and emotions I wrote about Wilma.

I had released her from her duty.

I had acknowledged her dedication to me.

I had given her permission to retire.

I was astounded and awed by the power I had to not only to communicate with my body parts but also to be heard, understood, and acknowledged. I had the power to converse with my organs, and they responded. It was a mutual relationship.

This was an amazing discovery. During the autumn of 1999, I discovered once again that I had the unbelievable power to heal my body. I wanted to run out and tell the world, but in 1999, who would have listened?

I wanted to pick up the phone and tell Louise Hay how much her work had helped me. I wanted to say, "Louise, you are so right!" I wanted to share with her how she had influenced my life.

I continued to use my body chats for my own body.

Story Two: Conclusion

Ten years later, my beliefs were put to yet another test. Louise Hay was with me one more time.

It appears that the universe tests me every ten years. Have you noticed any pattern in the times you have been tested in your life?

Maybe the 2009 test was my final exam, or maybe I will be tested again in ten years. If there is a pattern beyond every ten years, I have not identified it. I am sure when I turn 102, I will have arrived at the answer. I will be sure to Tweet you that one.

Sometimes I think I came to a fork in the road in 1989 and Louise Hay was standing there waiting to guide me down the healing path, for which I am most honored.

This healing path led me to becoming an energy healer. I am now a certified Emotional Freedom Technique (EFT) practitioner, a Matrix Reimprinting practitioner, and a life coach. I use the knowledge gained from Louise Hay on a daily basis to help and heal others.

Twenty Years after
Meeting Louise Hay

Fall 2009

In the autumn of 2009, I booked my yearly checkup at our local women's health clinic. I am big on regular checkups for both mammograms and pap smears. Although I sing the praises of natural healing, medical technology has so much to offer on the preventative side that we owe it to ourselves and our families to take advantage of these amazing devices and what they offer, namely early detection. We cannot self-heal what we are not aware exists. Early detection and self-healing complement one another.

The routine was normal. The attending female family doctor was informal enough to relax with but professional enough to make me feel confident. Just the balance I look for in professionals.

As she completed my internal examination, she expressed some concern about what she had just felt. The wall of my uterus was presenting as being thickened. I understood that at my then age of sixty-two, the uterus should have been thinning.

At her strong urging, I booked an ultrasound. Within two weeks, I was back to the local hospital for my ultrasound. The only ultrasound I had had up to that point was with my first pregnancy in 1970 when it was thought I might have been having twins. The ultrasound had cleared that up. I was having just one big, healthy boy.

The young technician was very professional and did a tremendous job at helping me feel comfortable. As she rotated the wand over my abdomen, she expressed some concern as to what she was seeing and asked if she could explore further for a more precise report. A more intrusive examination then followed.

Whether keeping within policy or out of human concern, the young woman pointed out on the screen what appeared to her to be a uterine abnormality. I dismissed this finding and headed home.

Not another thought entered my head about this until three days later when my phone rang. It was the doctor from the women's clinic who had strongly suggested I have an ultrasound. She informed me that my uterus had a thickening of the wall; a *thickened endometrium* I believe is the term she used. She indicated that this could be an indication of polyps, cysts, or even tumors. In other words, the wall was this thick for a reason, and it was not a positive one.

I was to contact my family doctor and get to a gynecologist as soon as possible. My appointment was set for late February 2010.

This was early November 2009, and it would be a three-month wait before I could see the specialist. I am a Canadian snowbird, which means as soon as the first flake of snow falls from the sky, usually mid-November, we head south to Florida, not to return until all snow has melted.

Keeping this appointment would mean flying back to Canada in February 2010 for a day and then back to Florida. I did some reflecting and informed my doctor that I had decided to wait until the spring for this appointment.

I told him I wanted to work on my self-healing, and this would give me six months to do so.

My family doctor offered all the necessary cautions and warnings involved with waiting the extra three months. I listened but stayed with my plan. The appointment was rescheduled for the last week of July, extending my self-healing time by an extra two months.

A cautionary note: I am not recommending deferring appointments with your doctor. Your life is precious and every second counts. But at that time, it felt like the right thing for me to do. I felt safe.

I was faithful to my daily body chats over the next eight months. Three times a day, I chatted with my uterus and its wall. Winter slipped into spring. Spring brought the snowbirds back north, and we headed home. Throughout those months, I communicated daily with Wilma. I strongly believed that I could correct whatever was wrong with my uterus.

During the winter of 2010, I began Emotional Freedom Technique (EFT) training with two of my now mentors in Florida. My healing now consisted of alternating my body chats with my EFT tapping. Both are forms of energy healing and seemed to complement each other nicely.

July came. My visit to a wonderful young gynecologist in July led to a biopsy to be followed by day surgery. The date was set for my hysteroscopy.

The health care I received was second to none. The gentleness, the professionalism, the one-on-one attention made our public system feel like a private clinic.

As I opened my eyes and started to come out of my anesthetic-induced sleep, the attending doctor shared with me his findings. To his amazement and somewhat mild disgust, he found a perfectly smooth-lined uterine wall.

I say he was amazed because the ultrasound report showed a different picture than what he had just witnessed and mild disgust because he felt that the ultrasound equipment must have been old or broken, and that this procedure was a waste not only of his time but also of public funds. He was, however, very gracious to me.

My follow-up appointment with him confirmed these feelings as he apologized for having put me through this procedure.

I so wanted to explain to this young doctor what really happened, that I healed myself, but his waiting room was filled with expectant mothers. It was July, and as most births occur in the month of September, these were very pregnant moms, and he was extremely busy.

In Retrospect

Even if I had the time to explain, I did not think that doctor was ready for the truth. Maybe one day. Not now. It was 2009.

What I would have told him was that there was nothing wrong with the ultrasound machine, the highly professional laboratory technician, or the doctor. They were all correct.

What I would have told him is that I healed myself. My body chats, directly speaking to my uterus wall and Wilma, combined with Louise Hay's healing method removed any unwanted whatever from my uterus, restoring it to one that was now healthy again.

Part I: Conclusion

Since these three major life-changing events, I feel I was put here to help others heal. The first lesson I learned from Louise Hay at the age of forty-two has influenced every part of my life. The process that evolved for me, body chats, has served me well. It was this mind-set that began in 1989 that has led me to Emotional Freedom Technique (EFT), of which I am at present a certified practitioner. Teaching others how to heal themselves has become an important part of my work.

Thank you, Louise Hay, for your major influence. Your work allowed me to develop into the healing person I am today.

May I always walk the healing path with you.

Each one of us is totally linked with the Universe and with all of life. The Power is within us to expand the horizons of our consciousness.

—Louise L. Hay

PART II

Self-Healing: How It Can Work for You

Healing

ဆဝဿ

The healing that I brought about in my own body was indeed amazing. Some might use the word *miracle* to describe what happened.

I was aware that it was a mind-body connection that made this work. But it was not until later that I came to understand the workings of the mind and body.

Shortly after my first healing, I began a master's degree in educational psychology and counseling. Nowhere in this intensive, full-time university program did I encounter any reference to self-healing. I guess at that time I basically tucked it away like any precious item in my life's treasure box.

Even though I once again used it in 1999, I did not go public with it. My healing remained a private event. It was not until my discovery of Emotional Freedom Technique (EFT) did I come to understand the workings of what I had achieved.

I truly believe that the universe works directly with us, but we have to be a cooperating partner. There is much for us to receive and enjoy, but we must be open. Our openness is our receptor for all that is good and possible in our world, all that the universe has to offer.

I mention openness as a lead into just how closed I was in my initial introduction to Emotional Freedom Technique. Actually, I was very cynical.

My introduction to Emotional Freedom Technique began in late September 2009. My oldest son, Sean, who you remember from his near-death experience, has been a well-established holistic trainer for over nineteen years and often shares with me some of his readings and intellectual findings. In late September 2009, I received an e-mail from him with the subject line: "You might find this interesting." The attachment read, "EFT video file."

I opened the file. In front of me was a person tapping on parts of his upper body. I watched, listened, and exited with the thought, *What is Sean into now? This is weird.*

About a month later, I was asked to present a short workshop to businesswomen in my geographical area. This success workshop was to be based on my first book, *Life Coaching Activities & Powerful Questions,* which was still in proof stage at that time. I prepared my workshop in detail, but several hours prior to presenting, I found I was getting a little anxious. An uncomfortable feeling started growing in my chest cavity. I was stepping outside my comfort zone in speaking to businesswomen. Thoughts like *What if the content of my book does not make sense?* and all the negative self-talk started flowing into my mind.

With only an hour to go, my thoughts immediately turned to that strange video my son had sent a month earlier. I went to my office, opened Sean's e-mail, and, yes, I started to tap. I tapped on the fear of public speaking.

I had a twenty-minute drive to the venue, and as I drove, I noticed that none of my usual anxiety over public speaking was surfacing. As I got closer to the building, I did a self-feelings check. Nothing. No anxiety. No tight feeling in my chest. *Surely it will arise as I enter a room of complete strangers, very busy businesswomen hoping for nuggets of wisdom from this life coach,* I thought.

I entered the room without an anxious thought or feeling. The two-hour presentation was well received, and I made new contacts. It was not until

I was halfway home on a dark country road that I became aware I was not anxious the whole evening. Could it be? Was it possible that a short time of tapping on points of my body released my anxiety? Not possible. I thought there must be another explanation.

Early one morning the following January, as I was doing my daily checking on LinkedIn, I noticed an announcement for EFT training in Orlando, Florida, just a short ride from my winter home. So I registered.

I openly admit that I approached this training with some degree of cynicism. But to my surprise, this dissipated quickly as one of the trainers, now my mentor, freed me from my fifty-year fear of dogs.

I have not looked back when it comes to EFT. I am now a certified practitioner and continue my studies in that area. It is a tool I offer my clients, and I personally use it daily to bring balance to my body and mind.

Throughout my training and continuous learning in the area of energy healing, I have come to understand that certain concepts and skills need to be present for self-healing to occur:

- belief that healing self is possible
- an open mind-set to the universe, the source, God
- intention, instilling within yourself a complete and deep sense that you want to be healed

Belief, Mind-set, and Intention

Belief, mind-set, and intention are necessary for self-healing. They must be present to create the mind-body connection. Please remember as you read this that I am not trained in metaphysics. I have a master's in educational psychology/counseling and am a certified Emotional Freedom Technique (EFT) practitioner. My understanding, knowledge, and skills come from a combination of my personal experiences, education, and training.

Belief

ເວດຕາ

We must believe in belief itself for it to have power in our lives.
—Greg Braden

Belief and My Early Years

My personal experiences in the area of formalized religion—at least perceived by me, and is it not our perceptions that become our reality?—focused much on belief and believing. As a young Catholic girl, I was never sure what I was to believe or have belief in. The teachings of the church, yes, but the word *believe* played a major role in my development.

The word was everywhere in the teachings, sermons, and lectures. "Believe and be saved," I heard continuously. The word *believe* was everywhere. But what did it mean? I struggled with this as a young girl. Many times, I wondered if my friends felt the same, but I was fearful to ask, as I might be committing a sin. So I tried my best to believe yet still not sure just what it was I was to believe in.

During my formative years of six and seven, I believed in Santa and was taught to believe in God. By nine, I was told there was no Santa, a belief I wanted to hold on to, but it was gone. I continued to believe in God for fear of spending an eternity in hell. I truly struggled as a young child with some of these beliefs, and fear filled many nightly thoughts.

41

I have always been fascinated by architectural designs. Back in the early sixties in my teen years, I passed this magnificent stone Protestant church daily on my way to school. I so wanted to see what this amazing structure looked like inside, but I believed that if I did, I would suffer a cruel fate to a Catholic—excommunication, expelled from the church and forever doomed, a lost soul roaming somewhere unknown.

These teachings of the church all changed in the mid-1960s with the twenty-first Ecumenical Council of the Catholic Church. While these changes were good, they led to much confusion for me as a young teenage girl. How could something that was true three years prior with such severe consequences now be dismissed? That belief was now shattered. As most young people did, I thought beliefs were based on facts.

That was the tipping point for my beginning to question the concept of belief and the implications related to any and all beliefs.

As if I needed a concrete example of how I was dealing with long-held beliefs, I watched as the amazing old gray-stone church came tumbling down piece by piece to make way for a road. The new regulations passed on from the Ecumenical Council came too late for me to see the inside of Saint Mary's Church.

In more recent times, the word *believe*, in every font possible, can be seen on items ranging from coffee mugs, t-shirts, and beach stones to wall murals.

But what does it mean?

How are we to interpret its meaning?

Is it belief in something unknown or unseen?

Is it belief in the supernatural?

Is it an unknown belief that we are expected to develop for reasons of faith?

Is it belief in the product being sold?

Belief and Personal Power

The belief I will address in this book is belief in your own personal power. It is belief in yourself and the ability you possess. It is also the set of supposed facts you have developed throughout your lifetime that structure that belief in your self.

Sometimes I think that the teachings and all the talk about belief I heard in church as a child was intended to achieve self-belief and self-love. I was raised a Christian, but I think all the great prophets understood fully the connection between our mind, body, and the universe. Through their words of wisdom, it was self-belief they wanted us to achieve. Had I been told that in my childhood, it would have made a lot more sense to me and would have indeed helped me at an earlier age with my personal success and understanding of our connectedness to the world.

I think the messages of the prophets were simple and designed to keep us happy, healthy, and at peace with one another and ourselves. This is what I now believe.

Your Beliefs

Your belief is how you think all the time based on what you understand to be fact. When you were a young child, depending on your culture, you, like me, may have believed there was a Santa Claus or some other fictional being. This was your belief based on what you perceived to be fact. As you got a little older, you came to understand that this belief was not fact but fiction. Your belief changed.

Much of how you react in and to the world and your daily events are based on your whole series of beliefs that started forming the second you were born or possibly even during gestation. In other words, much of what you think and believe and how you respond may have been similar to how your ancestors thought, believed, and behaved. Beliefs tend to be passed down from one generation to the next and oftentimes without being questioned, challenged, or changed.

Your beliefs hold much power for your health and happiness.

Your beliefs direct your life.

The beliefs that you hold may not be fact.

It is crucial that your beliefs be clarified and false ones deleted so you achieve maximum health and happiness.

Beliefs Can Change

Beliefs about our bodies come from many sources: family, friends, media, and culture. As with Santa Claus, these beliefs may not be fact, and yet they direct our lives.

Back in the early sixties, the TV show *Dragnet* featured a somewhat impatient but efficient homicide detective who had a classic line when speaking to witnesses, "Just the facts, ma'am. Just the facts."

Our beliefs may not be fact. If our beliefs are not serving us, we need to let them go and replace them with supportive beliefs. Just the facts ma'am.

Everything you think is not necessarily a belief.

When it comes to your health and healing your body, it is important to believe you can stay healthy. You must support this belief with words that encourage and nurture a healthy body.

My Healing

Some may view my healing as a miracle, and maybe it is. I guess it depends on your definition of a miracle. I now know my healing was a result of a combination of elements: the science of psychology, which includes the working of the subconscious mind; the universal power, the source, the field, God, whichever name you choose for your power source; and my belief in belief itself.

I believed the diseased cells would be replaced by healthy ones.

I believed in my recovery.

I believed I would get healthy.

I used words of support and spoke gently to my body as I would to one of my children.

In so doing, I brought my full awareness to the diseased cells in my body, focused on them, talked to them, and told them they were healthy. My attention for a period of time each day was directly centered on the cells of my body. Your energy flows where your attention goes.

My Questions

I am inquisitive by nature, and questions still float in my head around the process of my healing. You indeed may be asking the same questions as you read this book.

1. Did my direct focusing on and talking to my sick cells cause them to heal? Was it positive energy flowing where my attention was directed?
2. Was it that I believed I could heal that caused me to heal? Was it belief in my belief that healed me?

I am not a scientist and do not know the answers to these questions. But I do know that I healed myself, and that the combination of body chats and belief worked for me.

> In any project the important factor is your belief. Without belief there can be no successful outcome.
>
> —William James

Mind-set

ↂ

> Once your mindset changes, everything on the outside will
> change along with it.
>
> —Steve Maraboli

Your mind-set is your habitual way of thinking, feeling, and responding.
It consists of your beliefs, self-esteem, and level of persistence.

What Is Your Mind-set?

Here are a few questions to help you discover your personal mind-set:

How do you see the world?

What are your first thoughts when you get out of bed each morning?

Are they shaded with positive?

Are you a moaner-groaner in the mornings?

This is your mind-set. It is how you operate. Just like the operating system
of your computer, whether that be Windows or Apple, you have your own
operating system, your mind-set.

You can update your operating system (OS). The choice is yours.

In relation to this book and healing yourself, you need to take on the mindset that you can heal yourself. The more you use the healing activities in this book, the more you will feel your operating system shift.

Intention

৪০ ৫৪

Our intention creates our reality.

—Wayne Dyer

In the real-estate world, we always hear, "Location, location, location." In the self-healing world, it is intention, intention, intention.

Just what is this word *intention*? We hear it a lot at New Year's in relation to resolutions. Intention is purpose focused. Intention forms when you set your mind towards a project or desired goal.

Intention is what you plan to do based on a purpose you have in life. As you saw in my first story, my intention, my purpose in life, became to heal myself. I did not stop my regular daily routine, but my intention was so strong that I did not miss several times a day every day focusing on my intention, which was healing myself.

In recent times, research has been conducted around the power of intentions and its impact on personal health. The results have been positive.

When I use EFT in my practice, I help clients focus on their intention. I get them to focus on what they truly want to shift, change, or heal. I have found that tapping with deep intention leads to more successful and sustained results.

An intention synchronistically organizes its own fulfillment.
—Deepak Chopra

The Subconscious Mind

ಹಿ೦ಅ

Everything is energy and that's all there is to it. Match the frequency of the reality you want and you cannot help but get that reality. It can be no other way. This is not philosophy. This is physics.

—Albert Einstein

If I were to write about only one thing in this book, it would be the subconscious mind.

The subconscious mind directs 95 percent of your behavior, which means your conscious mind is involved in only 5 percent. What does this mean to you?

If you have been involved in self-development, no doubt you have heard all the quotes about your thinking and actions. Here are some of the most common:

Change your thinking and you'll change your world.
—Norman Peale

Our aspirations are our possibilities.
—Robert Browning

Your imagination is a preview of life's coming attractions.
—Albert Einstein

51

If you think you can or you can't, you're right.

—Henry Ford

In other words, your thoughts have a tremendous influence on your life, health, and success. They not only direct your actions, they also create them. You formulate your thinking into words to express yourself. Words, words, words influence your thinking.

Be careful with your words, for they get embedded in your subconscious mind and help create 95 percent of your actions, success, and health.

Watch Your P's and Q's

I often heard this expression from my parents when I was a teenager as I was heading out to visit friends or to just hang out: Mind your p's and q's. I knew what it meant for me, and although I had no idea of the origin of the p's and q's, I understood my parents were telling me to behave myself.

This phrase comes from a task performed by a bartender in British pubs. A chalkboard sat above the bar in the pub, and the tender would keep a tab of the punter's (bar patron's) drinks. As the drinks came in pints and quarts, the punter was reminded to watch his or her p's and q's. This phrase took on the broader translation of behaving yourself, the assumption being if you had too many p's and q's, your behavior may become somewhat inappropriate.

You literally need to watch your p's and q's and all the other twenty-four letters of the alphabet, as they form words in your thinking and leave your lips. These words will influence your behavior perhaps not in the same manner as the patrons of the pub, but maybe in even more personally devastating ways.

Every word you think or speak becomes embedded in your subconscious mind. First, you think. Second, you say the word. Then the word becomes embedded in your subconscious mind. It is extremely important to note that the subconscious mind takes everything literally.

Many of us grew up in cultures where some words became everyday language, and we now give no thought to how these words affect our thoughts and behavior and eventually our lives, successes, and health.

We are all familiar with the saying, "You are what you eat." Well, I believe you are also what you speak. Speaking is your thoughts verbalized. So be careful what you say. When you use negative words and phrases to describe yourself, predict your workday, or comment on any aspect of your life, the subconscious mind is listening.

The major role of your subconscious mind is to keep you safe. If you were bitten by a dog when you were young, chances are when you encountered a dog later in life, you moved away from it quickly. Your subconscious mind said, "Dog! Danger! Run!"

The subconscious mind listens to everything you think and say and programs it as fact.

Have you ever said, "I'm not lucky. If I didn't have bad luck, I'd have no luck at all"? The subconscious hears "not lucky" and will continue fulfilling what you say because it reads this message as what you want.

Your subconscious mind is like a computer, and you are the computer programmer. Every thought you have ever had and every word you have ever spoken is programmed into your subconscious mind as fact. The subconscious mind takes everything literally.

You are, in other words, creating your future self with every word you speak and every thought you think. So, again, be very careful what you say. In the words of W. Clement Stone: "You affect your subconscious mind by verbal repetition."

Words and Health

Just as your words create your future, they also contribute to your body's health and wellness.

The good news is that you can change those negative thoughts and beliefs. You can heal yourself through positive talk. You can heal yourself through body chats. Remember, the role of the subconscious mind is to keep you safe, so it will do as you say.

It is most important to your health that you rid yourself of the common language that has for some of us become a way of speaking to our bodies and our self. These negative conversations need to be changed if you are to have a happy, healthy life. The following are some common examples of negative self-talk:

- I am so stupid.
- My hair is always a mess.
- I can't remember a thing.
- I'm useless at math, computers, cooking, parenting, relationships, socializing, etc.
- I'll never be happy.
- I'll never have money.
- I know I'll die young. Everyone else in my family did.

The subconscious mind is now programmed by this negative self-talk, and this is the result: You will remain stupid with messy hair and not able to remember a name or date. You will not only be terrible at cooking, but you will also continue to be unhappy without a cent in your pocket and die young like the rest of your family. And you have created this version of you! Your subconscious mind takes this information, programs it as fact, and helps you live up to your beliefs. So ask yourself: Are these negative thoughts you have about yourself fact or fiction? Is this negative talk really true?

Your subconscious mind is also very willing to program your positive thoughts and language to turn your life around and make it the best it can be. It may take some time and practice to change your words to those that are positive and supportive, but you can do it. Your life may depend on it!

The subconscious mind can be your best friend or worst enemy. The good news is you get to choose which it will be.

It is time for you to make the change to a healthy and happier you.

Part II: Conclusion

Belief, intention, mind-set, and subconscious mind all come together in the process of self-healing.

To self-heal you must:

- believe you can heal yourself
- have a positive mind-set about your healing process
- have the intention to heal deep within your thoughts
- feed the subconscious mind with positive words and thoughts

Even though I healed myself and had a general idea as to how this happened—I talked to my body, and it listened—I did not truly understand the process within my body until I began my studies in energy healing. I now know that each and every one of us has been given the power to heal if we believe we can.

In Part Three, I offer you both preventative body chats and healing body chats, which will help you learn a new way to speak to your body.

PART III

Body Chats: Scripts for Self-Healing

Hold yourself as a mother holds her beloved child.

—The Buddha

The body chats I have developed and use are, for me, like a flower that has grown from the seed planted by Louise Hay.

In this section, I offer you the actual scripts I used to heal myself. I present them in both a preventative and a healing format. Depending on where you are on the health continuum, you may choose one or the other or both.

Preventative body chats and healing body chats will help you learn a new way to speak to your body and improve your health.

Treat your body lovingly, and it will respond in kind. Every word you think or speak becomes embedded in your subconscious mind. Make your words and thoughts be those of health and healing.

Body chats are a self-help tool and like any tool only work when used.

You Are Your Body

How do you speak to your best friend? Try using that same conversational style with any and all of your body parts. Do not ignore them. Chat with them daily. Be proactive in your health.

I always say to my clients that these are my words. But your body knows best. If while doing these activities another word or phrase you think best suits you comes to mind, please use it! As I said, your body knows best.

Preparation for Body Chats

In preparation for your body chats, please complete the following three steps. They are essential to preparing your mind and body for the amazing healing you are going to bring about. You have the power.

This preparation will allow your body to adjust your mind-set and focus your intention.

Step One: Your Healing Space

Set aside time and a quiet, comfortable space where you will not be interrupted. It does not have to be an elaborate setting, but it must be your space for the time you allot. This will be your healing space.

You are your body. Your body is not a piece of furniture or another inanimate object. Your body is an alive, dynamic, multiple-cell organ functioning continuously to bring you life energy. It *is* energy. Be kind to it, and you will receive many years of health and happiness.

Step Two: The Healing Light

All the power you need to heal comes from the universe, the source, the power, nature, God. Despite the title you choose, the power to heal is available if you ask.

See this power as a brilliant color, any color you choose, your favorite color if you like. I always use a golden light.

Bring this energy in the form of a brilliantly colored light into the crown of your head and have it flow through your body until it gets to the body part/organ you want to heal or keep healthy.

Surround the organ/body part with this brilliantly colored universal light, and observe as the organ/body part becomes strong and healthy. Visualize the disappearance of the red, raw, diseased parts and their replacement with healthy, strong cells.

Step Three: Body Chats

Greet this organ as you would your best friend. Tell it you have come to make it healthy and strong. Tell it you will be visiting it regularly from now on, and that you need its help in having a healthy and happy life.

Remember, you are working with energy that moves quickly. Just as you have the thought, the organ hears the message.

Begin your body chats for your brain, breasts, ears, eyes, nose, mouth, heart, lungs, stomach, legs, feet, arms, hands, and uterus. If you need to heal another body part, use existing scripts and insert the body part name.

Preventative Healing Body Chats and Activities

These scripts are designed in a proactive format so you can daily practice energy healing in the form of body chats. With each body chat, you bring the intention of health to your body parts.

My wish for you is that my body chats will help you have a healthy, happy life.

> If you have been diagnosed with a physical problem, disease, or illness, please be sure to follow your physician's orders with respect to medications, food, and exercise.

Brain Body Chat

Thank you, Brain, for all the functions you provide.

Without you where would I be?

You are my mainframe, my computer.

I am so happy that you have been with me since birth.

My memory is amazing.

I promise to exercise you more often with reading and mental activities.

You have helped me so much in my education and work. You are my source of wisdom.

You have been sending tweets and text messages to my body parts and muscles without fail. I thank you.

Activity

Place your hands on your head, and send vibrations of love and caring to your brain. See that love in a brilliant, vibrant color of your choosing. Have that vibrant color flow throughout your brain. Have it fill every cell in the right side and then the left side with this wonderful, healing energy.

Repeat three times: I love you, Brain, and thank you for all your work and dedication.

Breast Body Chats

I love you, Breasts.

You are a special part of me.

You provided a soft cushion for my babies to cuddle.

You offered nutrition to my babies.

I will keep you healthy.

Some have sexualized you, but that is not how I see you.

You are a part of my energy.

I will offer you support and care.

Your main biological function is to produce milk for babies, and I can accept this.

Activity

Place your hands on your breasts, and send vibrations of love and caring first to your right breast and then to your left breast. See that love in a brilliant, vibrant color of your choosing. Have that vibrant color flow throughout your right breast and then your left breast. Have it fill every cell in the right breast and then the left breast with this wonderful, healing energy.

Repeat three times: I love you, Breasts, and thank you for all your love and warmth.

Eyes Body Chat

Thank you, Eyes, for being my camera to the world.

Thank you, Eyes, for being my visual receptor to the world.

Eyes, you give me such joy in the amazing colors I see every day.

I love my (name color) eyes.

Eyes, you are strong and healthy.

Eyes, you allow me to navigate my world.

Eyes, you have helped me communicate with family and friends worldwide.

I will protect you from bright lights and glaring sun.

Activity

Place your hands on your eyes, and send vibrations of love and caring first to your right eye and then to your left eye. See that love in a brilliant, vibrant color of your choosing. Have that vibrant color flow throughout your right eye and then your left eye. Have it fill every cell in the right eye and then the left eye with this wonderful, healing energy.

Repeat three times: I love you, Eyes, and thank you for all your work and dedication.

Ears Body Chat

I love you, Ears!

You are my amazing stereo system.

You help me understand the spoken word.

Thank you for helping me to hear all the kind words of love and happiness.

You help me listen to everyone in my life.

You bring me pleasure from the wonderful sounds of music, rolling waves, my children's voices, and my parents' last words.

I will keep you safe and healthy.

Activity

Place your hands on your ears, and send vibrations of love and caring first to your right ear and then to your left ear. See that love in a brilliant, vibrant color of your choosing. Have that vibrant color flow throughout your right ear and then your left ear. Have it fill every cell in the right ear and then the left ear with this wonderful, healing energy.

Repeat three times: I love you, Ears, and thank you for all your work and dedication.

Nose Body Chat

I love you, Nose!

You warm the air and filter it as I breath.

You offer me happy memories of smells from the past, like my mom's cooking.

You warn me of certain dangers.

You refresh me with the wonderful aroma of spring flowers.

You may not be perfectly shaped, but you are my nose, and I accept you.

From the minute I was born, you allowed life's energy of oxygen to enter my lungs.

You hold my glasses as I read and write.

Activity

Place your hands on your nose, and send vibrations of love and caring to your nose. See that love in a brilliant, vibrant color of your choosing. Have that vibrant color flow throughout your right nostril and then your left nostril. Have it fill every cell in the nose with this wonderful, healing energy.

Repeat three times: *I love you, Nose, and thank you for all your work and dedication.*

Mouth Body Chat

I love you, Mouth.

You help me enjoy the delight of food.

I love how you let me express my opinion.

Thank you for giving me the ability to say, "I love you."

You allow me to pass smiles on to others.

You offer me the ability to enjoy and savor many amazing tastes.

You help process the nutrients as they enter my body.

You allow me to say kind words to others and to myself.

Activity

Place your hands on your mouth, and send vibrations of love and caring to your tongue, lips, and teeth. See that love in a brilliant, vibrant color of your choosing. Have that vibrant color flow into your mouth. Have it surround your tongue and teeth. Have it fill every cell in your mouth with this wonderful, healing energy.

Repeat three times: I love you, Mouth. Thank you for your work.

Heart Body Chat

I love you, Heart.

You are my source of life.

I can feel your wonderful rhythm as you pump, pump, pump the blood of life throughout my body. Thank you.

I need you to stay strong.

I love you and will exercise you often.

I will choose foods that will keep you healthy.

You have helped me feel joy. I now fill you with joy and happiness.

You are strong and healthy.

I need you every second of every day. You are my life source.

Activity

Place your hand on your heart. Feel its rhythm. Now visualize a brilliant, vibrant color of your choosing. Have this color fill your heart. Feel it, and see it move through each quadrant in your heart. Offer your heart your love and healing energy.

Repeat three times: I love you, Heart. I will always love you.

Lungs Body Chat

I love you, Lungs.

You are essential to my life.

You control every breath I take.

I can feel the wonderful air as it goes in and out of you.

You are amazing organs.

I promise to keep you healthy.

I need you to stay strong and healthy.

You have worked nonstop for me for _____ years. I owe you great health.

I need you, Lungs.

Activity

Place your hands on your lungs, and send vibrations of love and caring first to your left lung and then to your right lung. See that love in a brilliant, vibrant color of your choosing. Have that vibrant color flow into each lung. Have it fill every cell in your lungs with this wonderful, healing energy.

Repeat three times: I love you, Lungs. Thank you for your work.

Stomach Body Chat

I love you, Stomach.

Thank you for the work you do every day.

Sometimes I don't treat you as I should. I am sorry.

I promise I will be more kind to you in the future.

You are strong and healthy.

You digest my food with ease.

You will stay strong and health for years to come.

Stomach, you are very important in my life.

I love you, Stomach.

Activity

Place your hands on your stomach, and send vibrations of love and caring to every cell in your digestive system. See that love in a brilliant, vibrant color of your choosing. Have that vibrant color flow in and around your stomach. Visualize it filling every cell in your stomach with this wonderful, healing energy.

Repeat three times: I love you, Stomach. Thank you for your continuous work.

Legs and Feet Body Chat

Thank you, Legs and Feet. You are my support.

Legs and Feet, you are my transport system.

You help me run to safety.

You have helped me jump for joy.

You have taken me to many parts of the world.

Without you I wouldn't be able to explore the hilltops and valleys.

I send you love and accept you as you are.

I ask that you continue to support me as I move through each day, week, month, and year.

I promise to be more conscious of what you offer me.

Activity

Place your hands on your legs, and send vibrations of love and caring first to your hips and then all the way down to the tips of your toes. See that love in a brilliant, vibrant color of your choosing. Have that vibrant color flow down your left leg and into your left foot; now down your right leg and into your right foot. Have it fill every cell in your legs and feet with this wonderful, healing energy.

Repeat three times: I love you, Legs and Feet. Thank you for your support.

Arms and Hands Body Chat

I love you, Arms and Hands.

What could I do without you?

Hands, you held tightly to my parents when I was young.

Hands, you have touched the ones I love.

Hands, you have touched my dying parents, sending them my love.

Hands, you have been raised in protest for the rights of others.

Hands, you give me the ability to share the written word.

I now use you to help others heal and be happy.

Activity

Place your hands on your arms, and send vibrations of love and caring to your shoulders, arms, and hands. See that love in a brilliant, vibrant color of your choosing. Have that vibrant color flow downward, filling every cell in your shoulders, arms, and hands with this wonderful, healing energy.

Repeat three times: I love you, Arms and Hands. Thank you for embracing me.

Uterus Body Chat

I love you, Uterus.

You have been with me for many years.

You held/will hold my children.

You are strong and healthy.

You provide my body with needed hormones.

You are filled with potential.

I will be kinder to you from now on.

Thank you for what you offer.

You are very special to me.

Activity

Place your hands on the area of your uterus, and send vibrations of love and caring to this pear-shaped organ. See that love in a brilliant, vibrant color of your choosing. Have that vibrant color flow into your uterus. Have it fill every cell in your uterus with this wonderful, healing energy.

Repeat three times: I love you, Uterus. Thank you for being a part of me.

Healing Body Chat Scripts and Activities

I offer you energy-healing exercises in the form of body chats that you can practice daily. You will be sending positive words of healing to the ill organ/body part with the strong, heartfelt intention of healing, knowing you have the power within you to heal.

As you begin the body chats, you will visualize the organ or body part that has either been diagnosed with a health problem by a health care professional or is a source of pain or discomfort as you go about your daily life.

Note: If you have been diagnosed with a physical problem, disease, condition, or illness, please make sure you follow what your physician has prescribed with respect to medications, food, and exercise.

Preparation for Body Chats

In preparation for your body chats, please complete the following three steps. They are essential to preparing your mind and body for the amazing healing you are going to bring about. You have the power.

This preparation will allow your body to adjust your mind-set and focus your intention.

Three Steps of Preparation

Step One: Your Healing Space

Set aside time and a quiet, comfortable space where you will not be interrupted. It does not have to be an elaborate setting, but it must be your space for the time you allot. This will be your healing space.

You are your body. Your body is not a piece of furniture or another inanimate object. Your body is an alive, dynamic, multiple-cell organ functioning continuously to bring your life energy. It *is* energy. Be kind to it, and you will receive many years of health and happiness.

Step Two: The Healing Light

All the power you need to heal comes from the universe, the source, the power, nature, God. Despite the title you choose, the power to heal is available if you ask.

See this power as a brilliant color, any color you choose, your favorite color if you like. I always use a golden light.

Bring this energy in the form of a brilliantly colored light into the crown of your head and have it flow through your body until it gets to the body part/organ you want to heal or keep healthy.

Surround the body part/organ with this brilliant-colored universal light, and observe as the body part/organ becomes strong and healthy. Visualize the disappearance of the red, raw, diseased parts and their replacement with healthy, strong cells.

Step Three: Body Chats

Greet this organ as you would a best friend. Tell it you have come to make it healthy and strong. Tell it you will be visiting it regularly from now on, and that you need its help in having a healthy and happy life.

Remember, you are working with energy that moves quickly. Just as you have the thought, the organ hears the message.

Begin your body chats.

Heart Healing Body Chat

Visualize your heart.

Place your hand on your heart area.

Picture the problem area or diagnosis. See it as a red, raw area that is swollen and/or sore. You need to visualize the area that needs to be healed. Maybe it will mean seeing the heart fully.

Body Chat in Soft, Gentle Voice

I love you, Heart.

You are my source of life.

I need you to be healthy and strong.

The Healing Light

Now bring the healing light from the universe in the color you choose into the crown of your head, and have it move through your body to the area you want to heal. Talk to your heart as the color flows evenly and smoothly through every cell in your heart. See this brilliant-colored light encompass the diseased area. Visualize the redness being replaced by healthy cells.

Continue Your Body Chat

The healing is happening.

Redness, you are going and are being replaced by the healing light.

The redness is disappearing, the healing has started.

Heart, you are healthy. I can see you that way.

Heart, you are now strong and filled with healing light.

No more redness, no more disease. Healthy cells fill my heart.

My heart is strong and healthy.

I choose health.

I love you, Heart.

I need you, Heart.

You are my life.

I am healthy, and this is what I choose.

I can feel your steady beat.

You are healing.

Lungs Healing Body Chats

Visualize your lungs.

Place your hand on your lung area.

Picture the problem area or diagnosis. See it as a red, raw area that is swollen and/or sore. You need to visualize the area that needs to be healed.

Body Chat in Soft, Gentle Voice

I love you, Lung(s).

You are my source of life.

I need you to be healthy and strong.

The Healing Light

Now bring the healing light from the universe in the color you choose into the crown of your head, and have it move through your body to the area you want to heal. Talk to your lungs as the color flows evenly and smoothly through every cell in your lung(s). See this brilliant-colored light encompass the diseased area. Visualize the redness being replaced by healthy cells.

Continue Your Body Chat

The healing is happening.

Redness, you are going and are being replaced by the healing light.

The redness is disappearing, the healing has started.

Lungs, you are healthy. I can see you that way.

Lungs, you are now strong and filled with healing light.

No more redness, no more disease. Healthy cells fill my lungs.

My lungs are strong and healthy.

I choose health.

I love you, Lungs.

I need you, Lungs.

You are my life.

I am healthy, and this is what I choose.

I can feel your every breath.

You are healing.

Uterus Healing Body Chat

Visualize your uterus.

Place your hand on your uterine area.

Picture the problem area or diagnosis. See it as a red, raw area that is swollen and/or sore. You need to visualize the area that needs to be healed.

Body Chat in Soft, Gentle Voice

I love you, Uterus.

You are special to me.

I need you to be healthy and strong.

The Healing Light

Now bring the healing light from the universe in the color you choose into the crown of your head, and have it move through your body to the area you want to heal. Talk to your uterus as the color flows evenly and smoothly through every cell in your uterus. See this brilliant-colored light encompass the diseased area. Visualize the redness being replaced by healthy cells.

Continue Your Body Chat

The healing is happening.

Redness, you are going and are being replaced by the healing light.

The redness is disappearing, the healing has started.

Uterus, you are healthy. I can see you that way.

Uterus, you are now strong and filled with healing light.

No more redness, no more disease. Healthy cells fill my uterus.

Uterus, you are strong and healthy.

I choose health.

I love you, Uterus.

I need you, Uterus.

You are special in my life.

I am healthy, and this is what I choose.

I can feel your health returning.

You are healed.

Brain Healing Body Chat

Visualize your brain.

Place your hand on your head.

Picture the problem area or diagnosis. See it as a red, raw area that is swollen and/or sore. You need to visualize the area that needs to be healed.

Body Chat in Soft, Gentle Voice

I love you, Brain.

You are my source of understanding.

I need you to be healthy and strong.

The Healing Light

Now bring the healing light from the universe in the color you choose into the crown of your head, and have it move through your body to the area you want to heal. Talk to your brain as the color flows evenly and smoothly through every cell in the left side of your brain and then the right side of your brain. See this brilliant-colored light encompass the diseased area. Visualize the redness being replaced by healthy cells.

Continue Your Body Chat

The healing is happening.

Redness, you are going and are being replaced by the healing light.

The redness is disappearing; the healing has started.

Brain, you are healthy. I can see you that way.

Brain, you are now strong and filled with healing light.

No more redness, no more disease. Healthy cells fill my brain.

My brain is strong and healthy.

I choose health.

I love you, Brain.

I need you, Brain.

You guide me.

I am healthy, and this is what I choose.

I can feel your wisdom.

You are healing.

Stomach Healing Body Chat

Visualize your stomach.

Place your hand on your stomach area.

Picture the problem area or diagnosis. See it as a red, raw area that is swollen and/or sore. You need to visualize the area that needs to be healed.

Body Chat in Soft, Gentle Voice

I love you, Stomach.

You are my source of nutrition.

I need you to be healthy and strong.

The Healing Light

Now bring the healing light from the universe in the color you choose into the crown of your head, and have it move through your body to the area you want to heal. Talk to your stomach as the color flows evenly and smoothly through every cell in your stomach. See this brilliant-colored light encompass the diseased area. Visualize the redness being replaced by healthy cells.

Continue Your Body Chat

The healing is happening.

Redness, you are going and are being replaced by the healing light.

The redness is disappearing; the healing has started.

Stomach, you are healthy. I can see you that way.

Stomach, you are now strong and filled with healing light.

No more redness, no more disease. Healthy cells fill my digestive area.

My stomach is strong and healthy.

I choose health.

I love you, Stomach.

I need you, Stomach.

You are my life.

I am healthy, and this is what I choose.

I can feel you working for me.

You are healing.

Legs and Feet Healing Body Chat

Place your legs and feet in a position that is comfortable for you.

Picture the problem area or diagnosis. See it as a red, raw area that is swollen and/or sore. You need to visualize the area that needs to be healed.

Body Chat in Soft, Gentle Voice

I love you, Legs and Feet.

You are my source of transportation.

I need you to be healthy and strong.

The Healing Light

Now bring the healing light from the universe in the color you choose into the crown of your head, and have it move through your body to the area you want to heal. Talk to your legs and feet as the color flows evenly and smoothly through every cell from the top of your legs to the tips of your toes. See this brilliant-colored light encompass the diseased area. Visualize the redness being replaced by healthy cells.

Continue Your Body Chat

The healing is happening.

Redness, you are going and are being replaced by the healing light.

The redness is disappearing; the healing has started.

Legs and Feet, you are healthy. I can see you that way.

Legs and Feet, you are now strong and filled with healing light.

No more redness, no more disease. Healthy cells fill my legs and feet.

Legs and Feet, you are strong and healthy.

I choose health.

I love you, Legs and Feet.

I need you to move me forward.

You are my transportation system.

I am healthy, and this is what I choose.

I can feel your energy return. Legs and Feet, you are healthy.

You are healing.

Arms and Hands Healing Body Chat

Place your arms with hands resting in your lap. Make sure you are comfortable.

Picture the problem area or diagnosis. See it as a red, raw area that is swollen and/or sore. You need to visualize the area that needs to be healed.

Body Chat in Soft, Gentle Voice

I love you, Arms and Hands.

You are a part of everything I do.

I need you to be healthy and strong.

The Healing Light

Now bring the healing light from the universe in the color you choose into the crown of your head, and have it move through your body to the area you want to heal. Talk to your arms and hands as the color flows evenly and smoothly through every cell from the top of your legs to the tips of your toes. See this brilliant-colored light encompass the diseased area. Visualize the redness being replaced by healthy cells.

Continue Your Body Chat

The healing is happening.

Redness, you are going and are being replaced by the healing light.

The redness is disappearing; the healing has started.

Arms and Hands, you are healthy. I can see you that way.

My arms and hands are now strong and filled with healing light.

No more redness, no more disease. My arms and hands are filled with strong, healthy cells.

Arms and Hands, you are strong and healthy.

I choose health.

I love you, Arms and Hands.

I need you for my daily activities.

I need you to help me hug others.

I am healthy, and this is what I choose.

I can feel your energy return. Arms and Hands, you are healthy.

You are healed.

Eyes Healing Body Chat

Place your hand on your eyes.

Visualize the inside of your eyes.

Picture the problem area or diagnosis. See it as a red, raw area that is swollen and/or sore. You need to visualize the area that needs to be healed.

Body Chat in Soft, Gentle Voice

I love you, Eyes.

You are my camera on the world.

I need you to be healthy and strong.

The Healing Light

Now bring the healing light from the universe in the color you choose into the crown of your head, and have it move through your body to the area you want to heal. Talk to your eyes as the color flows evenly and smoothly through every cell in your left eye and then your right eye. See this brilliant-colored light encompass the diseased area. Visualize the redness being replaced by healthy cells.

Continue Your Body Chat

The healing is happening.

Redness, you are going and are being replaced by the healing light.

The redness is disappearing the healing has started.

Eyes, you are healthy.

Eyes, you are now strong and filled with healing light.

No more redness, no more disease. My eyes are filled with healthy cells.

My eyes are strong and healthy.

I choose health.

I love you (name color) eyes.

I need you, Eyes.

You are my lens on the world.

I am healthy, and this is what I choose.

I can feel energy/light returning. All is well.

You are healed.

Headache

Place your hands on the part of your head that hurts. See it as a red, raw area that is swollen and/or sore. You need to visualize the area that needs to be healed.

Body Chat in Soft, Gentle Voice

I love you, Head.

You are a part of everything I do.

I need you to be healthy and strong.

The Healing Light

Now bring the healing light from the universe in the color you choose into the crown of your head, and have it move to the painful area in your head. See the color flow evenly and smoothly, filling every cell in and around the pain. Talk to your head.

Continue Your Body Chat

The healing is happening.

Pain, you are going and are being replaced by the healing light.

The pain is disappearing; comfort is returning.

Head, you are healthy. I can see you that way.

The pain is leaving my head.

No more aches, no more discomfort.

Head, you are strong and healthy.

I choose a head without aches and pains.

I love you, Head.

I need you for a joyful day.

I need you to help me think.

The source of pain has left me.

I choose my days without headaches.

Head, I can feel your energy return.

My headache is gone.

Back Pain

Place your hand on the area of your back pain, or if that is uncomfortable for you, picture the painful spot. See it as a red, raw area that is swollen and/or sore. You need to visualize the area that needs to be healed.

Body Chat in Soft, Gentle Voice

I love you, (name location of pain).

You are a part of everything I do.

I need you to be healthy and strong.

The Healing Light

Now bring the healing light from the universe in the color you choose into the crown of your head, and have it move through your body to the painful area of your back. See the color flow evenly and smoothly, filling every cell in and around the pain. Talk to your back.

Continue Your Body Chat

The healing is happening.

Pain, you are going and are being replaced by the healing light.

The pain is disappearing; the healing has started.

Back, you are healthy. I can see you that way.

My back (upper/lower) is now strong and filled with healing light.

No more pain, no more stiffness. My back is filled with strong, healthy cells.

Back, you are strong and healthy.

I choose health.

I love you, Back.

I need you for my daily activities.

The source of pain is gone.

I choose my days without back pain.

I can feel your energy return.

There is no pain.

You are healed.

Part III: Conclusion

These body chats healed me and continue to keep me healthy.

I reprogrammed my subconscious mind so that it adjusted the sick cells within my body and created healthy cells as I asked.

I invite you to do the same.

We get one life to live, so why not make it the best it can be? Good health is one of the largest factors of a good life.

> Any thought that is passed on to the subconscious often
> enough and convincingly enough is finally accepted.
> —Robert Collier

About the Author

Phyllis E. Reardon M.Ed is a life coach, author, motivational speaker, and EFT practitioner. Phyllis has used her gift of intuition throughout her working life as a teacher and counselor to help others realize their potential. She has always been a helper. With the knowledge she gained from one little blue book, *Heal Your Body* by Louise L. Hay, she not only learned to self-heal but also uses this wisdom to help heal others.

Phyllis holds a B.A.Ed and M.Ed. Phyllis is also the author of *Life Coaching Activities & Powerful Questions* (2009), *Know Your Strengths Inventory* (2011), and *Life Coaching Questions* (2012).

Phyllis lives in Newfoundland and Labrador, Canada, and can be easily reached at phyllis@coachphyllis.com.

www.ingramcontent.com/pod-product-compliance
Lightning Source LLC
Chambersburg PA
CBHW030347290526
45785CB00004B/1634